# " The Power of Nutrition in Shaping Our Minds "

# INTRODUCTION

Harnessing the Potential for Optimal Mental Health." In this guide, we will delve into the remarkable influence of nutrition on our minds and explore how conscious choices about what we eat can have a transformative impact on our mental well-being.

In today's fast-paced world, where stress and mental health concerns are prevalent, it is essential to recognize the profound connection between what we consume and how it affects our minds. While we often associate nutrition with physical health, its influence extends far beyond that. Scientific research has increasingly highlighted the significant role that nutrition plays in shaping our mental health, cognitive function, emotional well-being, and overall resilience.

Throughout this ebook, we will uncover the intricate relationship between nutrition and mental health. We will explore the essential nutrients that support optimal brain function, such as omega-3 fatty acids,

B-vitamins, antioxidants, and minerals. Understanding the vital role of these nutrients empowers us to make informed choices about the foods we consume and their impact on our cognitive excellence.

Furthermore, we will examine the link between nutrition and emotional resilience, as certain micronutrients play a crucial role in regulating our mood and emotional well-being. We will explore the connection between our gut and our mind, unraveling the fascinating mind-gut axis and the importance of nurturing a healthy gut microbiome for mental harmony.

In addition, we will delve into the impact of inflammation on mental health and how adopting an anti-inflammatory diet can promote better mental well-being. We will shed light on the detrimental effects of processed foods and excessive sugar intake, providing strategies for reducing their consumption and embracing nutrient-dense alternatives.

Lastly, we will explore how optimal nutrition fuels mental performance, enhancing cognitive agility, memory, and concentration. By incorporating brain-boosting nutrients into our diets, we can unlock our cognitive potential and thrive in various aspects of our lives.

Join us on this enlightening journey as we uncover the power of nutrition in shaping our minds and embrace the opportunity to prioritize our mental well-being through conscious dietary choices. Together, let us harness the potential of nutrition for optimal mental health.

# INDEX

- Nourishing the Brain

- Emotional Resilience

- The Mind-Gut Connection

- Anti-Inflammatory Foods

- Managing Stress

- Healthy Fats for Brain Health

- Sustainable Nutrition for Long-term Well-being

- Gut-Brain Axis and Mental Health

- Lifestyle Factors and Mental Health

- The Impact of Processed Foods and Sugar on Mental Health

# Chapter 1

# Nourishing the Brain

Proper nutrition is essential for optimal brain function, as our brain requires a range of nutrients to perform at its best. In this section, we will delve into the essential nutrients that support brain health, including omega-3 fatty acids, B-vitamins, antioxidants, and minerals. Understanding the role of these nutrients and incorporating them into our diets can have a profound impact on our cognitive abilities, memory, and overall brain function.

Omega-3 fatty acids are crucial for brain health and development. They are particularly abundant in fatty fish like salmon, mackerel, and sardines. These fatty acids, specifically EPA and DHA, play a vital role in the structure and function of brain cells. They support the communication between brain cells, enhance cognitive abilities, and contribute to overall mental well-being. Incorporating omega-3-rich foods into our diets or considering supplements can be beneficial, especially for those who don't consume fish regularly.

B-vitamins, including thiamine, riboflavin, niacin, vitamin B6, vitamin B12, and folate, are essential for energy production, neurotransmitter synthesis, and overall brain function. They can be found in various food sources such as whole grains, legumes, leafy greens, eggs, and meat. B-vitamins are involved in processes that support memory, concentration, and cognitive performance. Ensuring an adequate intake of these vitamins through a balanced diet can contribute to optimal brain health.

Antioxidants, such as vitamin C, vitamin E, and various phytochemicals found in fruits and vegetables, play a crucial role in protecting our brain cells from oxidative stress and damage caused by free radicals. These compounds help reduce inflammation and support healthy brain aging. Consuming a variety of brightly colored fruits and vegetables, such as berries, citrus fruits, spinach, and kale, can provide a rich source of antioxidants.

Minerals, such as iron, zinc, magnesium, and copper, are vital for brain function and are involved in various processes, including neurotransmitter synthesis, oxygen transport, and energy production. Iron, for example, is necessary for oxygen supply to the brain, while zinc supports memory and learning. Good food sources of these minerals include lean meats, seafood, whole grains, nuts, and seeds. Incorporating these nutrient-rich foods into our diets ensures an adequate supply of essential minerals for optimal brain function.

In addition to these specific nutrients, adopting a balanced and varied diet that includes a wide range of fruits, vegetables, whole grains, lean proteins, and healthy fats is key to providing the necessary nourishment for the brain. A well-rounded diet ensures a diverse array of nutrients that work synergistically to support brain health and function.

It is important to note that while certain nutrients have been associated with improved cognitive function, memory, and overall brain health, they do not act in isolation. The overall dietary pattern and lifestyle factors, such as physical activity and stress management, also play significant roles in maintaining optimal brain health.

In summary, nourishing the brain involves understanding the importance of essential nutrients such as omega-3 fatty acids, B-vitamins, antioxidants, and minerals. These nutrients support brain function, enhance cognitive abilities, and contribute to overall mental well-being. By incorporating nutrient-rich foods into our diets and adopting a balanced eating pattern, we can provide our brains with the necessary nourishment for optimal performance and long-term brain health. Prioritizing brain-nourishing foods and embracing a healthy lifestyle can have a profound impact on our cognitive abilities, memory, and overall mental well-being.

# Chapter 2

**Emotional Resilience**

Emotional resilience refers to our ability to adapt, bounce back, and maintain a positive outlook in the face of adversity and stressful situations. It plays a crucial role in our overall mental well-being and quality of life. In this section, we will explore the connection between nutrition and emotional resilience, highlighting the importance of specific nutrients in promoting emotional well-being.

One of the key players in emotional resilience is serotonin, a neurotransmitter often referred to as the "feel-good" chemical. Serotonin helps regulate mood, emotions, and promotes a sense of well-being. Tryptophan, an amino acid found in various foods, is a precursor to serotonin production. Consuming tryptophan-rich foods, such as turkey, eggs, nuts, and seeds, can support the production of serotonin, thus enhancing emotional resilience.

Vitamin D, often called the "sunshine vitamin," is another essential nutrient for emotional well-being. It not only plays a role in bone health but also influences our mood and mental health. Low levels of vitamin D have been linked to an increased risk of depression and seasonal affective disorder (SAD). While our bodies can produce vitamin D when exposed to sunlight, dietary sources such as fatty fish, fortified dairy products, and eggs can contribute to maintaining optimal vitamin D levels.

Magnesium, known for its calming properties, is a mineral that supports emotional resilience. It helps regulate stress responses, relaxes muscles, and promotes a sense of calmness. Good food sources of magnesium include leafy greens, nuts, seeds, whole grains, and legumes. Incorporating these foods into our diets can contribute to emotional well-being and stress management.

Zinc, an essential trace mineral, is involved in numerous biochemical processes in the body, including neurotransmitter function and mood regulation. Low levels of zinc have been associated with an increased risk of depression and anxiety. Foods rich in zinc include oysters, shellfish, lean meats, legumes, seeds, and nuts. By including these foods in our diet, we can support emotional resilience and mental well-being.

In addition to specific nutrients, adopting a well-balanced diet that includes a variety of whole foods, such as fruits, vegetables, whole grains, lean proteins, and healthy fats, is crucial for emotional resilience. These foods provide a range of nutrients, antioxidants, and phytochemicals that work synergistically to support our overall mental health.

It's important to note that while nutrition is a significant factor in emotional resilience, it is just one piece of the puzzle. Other lifestyle factors, such as regular physical activity, sufficient sleep, stress management techniques, and social connections, also contribute to emotional well-being.

In summary, emotional resilience is vital for navigating the challenges of life and maintaining positive mental health. Nutrition plays a crucial role in promoting emotional resilience by providing the body with essential nutrients that support mood regulation and overall emotional well-being. Incorporating tryptophan-rich foods, ensuring adequate vitamin D levels, consuming magnesium and zinc-rich foods, and adopting a well-balanced diet are key strategies for enhancing emotional resilience. By prioritizing our nutrition and embracing a holistic approach to mental well-being, we can cultivate emotional resilience and thrive in the face of adversity.

# Chapter 3

## The Mind-Gut Connection

The mind-gut connection refers to the bidirectional communication network between the brain and the gut. It highlights the influence of the gut microbiota, the community of microorganisms residing in our digestive tract, on our mental health, emotions, and overall well-being. In this section, we will explore the fascinating mind-gut connection and how nurturing a healthy gut microbiome can positively impact mental health.

The gut is often referred to as our "second brain" due to the complex network of neurons lining the gastrointestinal tract, known as the enteric nervous system. This intricate system communicates with the central nervous system, which includes the brain, via various pathways, including neural, hormonal, and immune mechanisms. This bidirectional communication enables constant information exchange between the gut and the brain, influencing both physical and mental health.

The gut microbiota, consisting of trillions of bacteria, viruses, fungi, and other microorganisms, plays a significant role in the mind-gut connection. These microorganisms contribute to vital functions such as digestion, nutrient absorption, and immune system regulation. They also produce neurotransmitters and other molecules that can influence brain function and behavior.

Research has shown a strong association between the composition of the gut microbiota and mental health conditions such as anxiety, depression, and stress. Imbalances in the gut microbiome, known as dysbiosis, have been linked to increased susceptibility to mental health disorders. On the other hand, a diverse and healthy gut microbiota is associated with improved mental well-being and resilience.

Nurturing a healthy gut microbiome involves adopting dietary and lifestyle practices that promote the growth of beneficial bacteria. Consuming a diet rich in fiber from fruits, vegetables, whole grains, and legumes provides prebiotic fibers that serve as food for beneficial gut bacteria. These fibers help stimulate the growth of beneficial species and support a diverse and thriving gut microbiota.

Probiotics, live bacteria that confer health benefits when consumed, can also contribute to a healthy gut microbiome. Fermented foods like yogurt, kefir, sauerkraut, and kimchi are natural sources of probiotics.

Probiotic supplements are also available and can be beneficial in restoring and maintaining a balanced gut microbiota.

Furthermore, reducing the intake of processed foods, artificial additives, and excessive sugar can help maintain a healthy gut microbiome. These dietary factors can negatively impact the diversity and balance of gut bacteria, leading to dysbiosis and potential negative effects on mental health.

In addition to dietary strategies, lifestyle factors such as regular exercise, adequate sleep, stress management, and avoiding unnecessary antibiotic use can also contribute to a healthy gut microbiome and support the mind-gut connection. Exercise has been shown to positively influence the diversity and composition of gut bacteria, while chronic stress can disrupt the delicate balance of the gut microbiota.

Understanding the mind-gut connection opens up new avenues for interventions in mental health. Emerging research suggests that strategies aimed at modulating the gut microbiota, such as probiotics, prebiotics, and fecal microbiota transplantation (FMT), hold promise in improving mental health outcomes. However, further research is needed to fully understand the complex mechanisms underlying the mind-gut connection and develop targeted therapies.

In summary, the mind-gut connection highlights the intricate relationship between our gut microbiota, the gut-brain axis, and mental health.

Nurturing a healthy gut microbiome through a balanced diet rich in fiber, probiotic foods, and reducing the intake of processed foods can positively impact mental well-being. By prioritizing our gut health, we can harness the power of the mind-gut connection and potentially improve our mental health and overall well-being.

# Chapter 4

**Anti-Inflammatory Foods**

Inflammation is a natural response of the body to injury or infection. However, chronic inflammation can contribute to various health issues, including cardiovascular disease, diabetes, and autoimmune disorders. In this section, we will explore the concept of anti-inflammatory foods and how incorporating them into our diets can help reduce inflammation and promote better overall health.

Anti-inflammatory foods are those that possess properties that help counteract inflammation in the body. They are rich in antioxidants, phytochemicals, and essential nutrients that have been shown to reduce inflammatory markers and promote a balanced immune response.

One key group of anti-inflammatory foods is fruits and vegetables, particularly those with vibrant colors. Berries, leafy greens, tomatoes, and citrus fruits are abundant in antioxidants, including vitamins C and E, which help neutralize free radicals and reduce oxidative stress. These antioxidants also possess anti-inflammatory properties that can support the body's natural defense against inflammation.

Healthy fats, such as those found in avocados, nuts, seeds, and fatty fish like salmon, are another important component of an anti-inflammatory diet. These foods are rich in omega-3 fatty acids, specifically eicosapentaenoic acid (EPA) and docosahexaenoic acid (DHA), which have potent anti-inflammatory effects. Omega-3 fatty acids help balance the body's inflammatory response by reducing the production of pro-inflammatory molecules.

Whole grains, such as brown rice, quinoa, and whole wheat bread, are also valuable additions to an anti-inflammatory diet. They provide a good source of fiber and other nutrients that support a healthy gut microbiota. A diverse and thriving gut microbiome has been linked to reduced inflammation and improved overall health.

Herbs and spices like turmeric, ginger, garlic, and cinnamon possess powerful anti-inflammatory properties. Turmeric, in particular, contains curcumin, a compound renowned for its potent anti-inflammatory effects. Adding these herbs and spices to our meals not only enhances the flavor but also boosts the anti-inflammatory potential of our diets.

Legumes, such as lentils, chickpeas, and beans, are excellent sources of plant-based protein, fiber, and other nutrients. They offer a wide array of antioxidants and phytochemicals that can combat inflammation and promote a healthy immune system.

Incorporating legumes into our meals provides us with a nutritious and anti-inflammatory plant-based protein option.

In contrast, highly processed and refined foods, including sugary snacks, fried foods, and refined carbohydrates, can promote inflammation in the body. These foods are often high in added sugars, unhealthy fats, and artificial additives, which can trigger an inflammatory response. Limiting the consumption of these inflammatory foods is crucial for maintaining optimal health.

Adopting an anti-inflammatory diet involves making conscious choices to prioritize whole, unprocessed foods and reducing the intake of inflammatory triggers. By incorporating a variety of fruits, vegetables, healthy fats, whole grains, herbs, and spices into our meals, we can provide our bodies with the necessary nutrients and compounds to combat inflammation and promote overall well-being.

It is important to note that while an anti-inflammatory diet can be beneficial, it is just one component of a healthy lifestyle. Regular physical activity, stress management, and adequate sleep are also vital for reducing inflammation and maintaining optimal health.

In summary, an anti-inflammatory diet focuses on incorporating foods rich in antioxidants, phytochemicals, and essential nutrients that help reduce inflammation in the body. Including fruits, vegetables, healthy fats, whole grains, legumes, herbs, and spices while limiting processed and inflammatory foods can support a balanced immune response and promote overall well-being. By adopting an anti-inflammatory diet and embracing a holistic approach to health, we can take proactive steps towards reducing inflammation and improving our long-term health outcomes.

# Chapter 5

**Managing Stress**

Stress has become an unavoidable part of modern life, and chronic stress can have detrimental effects on our physical and mental well-being. However, by understanding the underlying mechanisms of stress and implementing effective stress management strategies, we can mitigate its impact on our lives. In this section, we will explore various approaches to managing stress and promoting a healthier, more balanced lifestyle.

Firstly, it's essential to recognize the signs and symptoms of stress. Stress can manifest in physical symptoms such as headaches, muscle tension, and digestive issues, as well as emotional and cognitive symptoms such as irritability, anxiety, and difficulty concentrating. Being aware of these indicators allows us to identify stressors and take proactive steps to manage them.

One effective strategy for managing stress is adopting relaxation techniques. Deep breathing exercises, meditation, and mindfulness practices help activate the body's relaxation response, reducing the physiological and psychological effects of stress. Regular practice of these techniques can promote a sense of calmness and improve overall well-being.

Physical activity plays a significant role in stress management. Engaging in regular exercise releases endorphins, known as "feel-good" hormones, which boost mood and reduce stress levels. Activities such as walking, jogging, yoga, or any form of exercise that you enjoy can be beneficial in managing stress. Finding ways to incorporate physical activity into our daily routines is essential for long-term stress reduction.

A balanced diet is crucial for both physical and mental well-being. Certain foods can help regulate stress levels and promote relaxation. Consuming complex carbohydrates, such as whole grains and legumes, can increase the production of serotonin, a neurotransmitter that enhances mood. Foods rich in omega-3 fatty acids, such as fatty fish, walnuts, and flaxseeds, have been shown to reduce symptoms of stress and anxiety. Additionally, ensuring adequate intake of vitamins and minerals through a diverse diet supports optimal brain function and stress management.

Effective time management is another key aspect of stress management. Prioritizing tasks, setting realistic goals, and practicing effective time allocation can help reduce feelings of being overwhelmed. Breaking larger tasks into smaller, manageable chunks and establishing a structured routine can enhance productivity and reduce stress levels.

Social support is essential in managing stress. Sharing our feelings and experiences with trusted friends, family members, or support groups can provide emotional comfort and a sense of belonging. Engaging in meaningful social connections, whether through personal interactions or joining community activities, helps reduce feelings of isolation and promotes a support system during challenging times.

Taking regular breaks and engaging in activities we enjoy is vital for stress reduction. Engaging in hobbies, spending time in nature, listening to music, or practicing creative outlets can provide a sense of relaxation and help shift our focus away from stressors. Incorporating these activities into our daily routines allows for regular moments of rejuvenation and enjoyment.

Managing stress also involves setting boundaries and practicing self-care. Learning to say no to excessive commitments, delegating tasks, and prioritizing self-care activities such as getting enough sleep, practicing good hygiene, and engaging in activities that promote relaxation and personal well-being are crucial for managing stress effectively.

Additionally, stress management techniques can be complemented by professional help. Seeking support from therapists, counselors, or psychologists can provide valuable guidance and strategies for coping with stress. They can help identify underlying causes of stress and offer tailored approaches for managing specific stressors.

In summary, managing stress involves adopting a holistic approach that encompasses relaxation techniques, physical activity, a balanced diet, effective time management, social support, leisure activities, setting boundaries, and self-care practices. By incorporating these strategies into our daily lives, we can reduce the negative impact of stress and promote overall well-being. It is important to remember that managing stress is an ongoing process, and it may require experimentation to find the most effective combination of techniques that work for each individual.

## Chapter 6

### Healthy Fats for Brain Health

The brain is a complex organ that requires proper nutrition to function optimally. Healthy fats play a crucial role in supporting brain health and cognitive function. In this section, we will explore the importance of healthy fats and highlight specific types of fats that are beneficial for the brain.

Omega-3 fatty acids are a type of polyunsaturated fat that are essential for brain health. They are particularly important for the development and maintenance of brain cells and the nervous system. Two types of omega-3 fatty acids, eicosapentaenoic acid (EPA) and docosahexaenoic acid (DHA), have been extensively studied for their positive effects on brain function.

DHA, in particular, is a major structural component of the brain and is vital for proper brain development in infants and children. It supports cognitive function, memory, and learning throughout life. EPA, on the other hand, is involved in reducing inflammation and promoting overall brain health.

Fatty fish, such as salmon, mackerel, sardines, and trout, are excellent sources of omega-3 fatty acids. Consuming these fish regularly can provide an abundant supply of DHA and EPA to support brain health. For those who do not consume fish, algae-based supplements are available as an alternative source of omega-3 fatty acids.

In addition to fatty fish, other foods rich in healthy fats can also benefit brain health. Avocados are an excellent source of monounsaturated fats, which support healthy blood flow and provide essential nutrients to the brain. They also contain vitamin E, an antioxidant that helps protect brain cells from oxidative damage.

Nuts and seeds, such as walnuts, almonds, flaxseeds, and chia seeds, are packed with healthy fats, including omega-3 fatty acids, monounsaturated fats, and polyunsaturated fats. These fats provide essential nutrients and antioxidants that support brain health. Including a variety of nuts and seeds in our diet can help enhance cognitive function and protect against age-related cognitive decline.

Olive oil, a staple in the Mediterranean diet, is rich in monounsaturated fats and has been associated with numerous health benefits, including improved brain health. Its antioxidant properties help reduce inflammation and oxidative stress in the brain, promoting better cognitive function and protecting against neurodegenerative diseases.

Coconut oil, although high in saturated fats, contains medium-chain triglycerides (MCTs) that are metabolized differently in the body. MCTs are a source of quick energy for the brain and have been studied for their potential cognitive benefits. However, further research is needed to fully understand their impact on brain health.

It's important to note that while healthy fats are beneficial for brain health, they should be consumed in moderation as part of a balanced diet. Portion control is key to maintaining a healthy weight and preventing the negative effects of excessive calorie intake.

In summary, healthy fats play a vital role in supporting brain health and cognitive function. Omega-3 fatty acids, particularly DHA and EPA, are essential for brain development, memory, and overall brain health. Fatty fish, such as salmon, are excellent sources of these omega-3 fatty acids. Additionally, avocados, nuts, seeds, olive oil, and coconut oil are rich in healthy fats that can support brain function. By incorporating these foods into our diet and maintaining a balanced approach to fat consumption, we can provide our brains with the essential nutrients they need to thrive.

# Chapter 7

## Sustainable Nutrition for Long-term Well-being

Sustainable nutrition is a holistic approach to eating that promotes not only personal health but also the health of the planet. It emphasizes the consumption of whole, minimally processed foods while considering the environmental impact of our dietary choices. In this section, we will explore the concept of sustainable nutrition and its benefits for long-term well-being.

One of the key principles of sustainable nutrition is focusing on plant-based foods. Plant-based diets, such as vegetarian or vegan diets, have been associated with numerous health benefits, including reduced risk of chronic diseases such as heart disease, obesity, and certain types of cancer. These diets also tend to have a lower carbon footprint compared to diets rich in animal products.

Including a variety of fruits, vegetables, whole grains, legumes, nuts, and seeds in our diets provides us with essential nutrients, fiber, and antioxidants that support optimal health. These plant-based foods are generally more sustainable to produce and require fewer resources compared to animal-based products.

Another important aspect of sustainable nutrition is reducing food waste. Food waste not only contributes to environmental issues such as greenhouse gas emissions but also represents a significant loss of valuable resources. Planning meals, storing food properly, and being mindful of portion sizes can help minimize food waste and promote a more sustainable approach to nutrition.

Choosing locally sourced and seasonal foods is another pillar of sustainable nutrition. Buying produce from local farmers reduces transportation-related emissions and supports the local economy. Seasonal foods are often fresher, tastier, and more nutritious, as they are harvested at their peak and require fewer artificial inputs to grow.

Sustainable nutrition also encourages mindful eating practices. Taking the time to savor and appreciate our meals can help us develop a healthier relationship with food and make more conscious choices. Mindful eating involves listening to our body's hunger and fullness cues, eating slowly, and being aware of the flavors and textures of the foods we consume.

Incorporating sustainable protein sources into our diets is essential for long-term well-being. While animal-based proteins can be part of a sustainable diet, choosing alternatives such as legumes, tofu, tempeh, and seitan can significantly reduce our environmental impact. These plant-based proteins are not only rich in nutrients but also require fewer resources to produce.

Reducing the consumption of highly processed foods and prioritizing whole, unprocessed foods is another key aspect of sustainable nutrition. Processed foods often contain additives, preservatives, and excessive amounts of salt, sugar, and unhealthy fats. Opting for whole foods not only supports our health but also reduces packaging waste and the carbon footprint associated with food processing.

Sustainable nutrition is closely linked to sustainable agriculture practices. Supporting organic farming methods, regenerative agriculture, and small-scale farmers helps promote biodiversity, soil health, and sustainable food production. Choosing organic produce and supporting local, sustainable food systems can contribute to a healthier planet and long-term well-being.

Educating ourselves about the impact of our food choices is an integral part of sustainable nutrition. By staying informed about food labels, certifications, and understanding the environmental implications of different farming practices, we can make more informed decisions and actively support sustainable food systems.

In summary, sustainable nutrition encompasses a range of practices that promote long-term well-being for both individuals and the planet. By focusing on plant-based foods, reducing food waste, choosing local and seasonal produce, practicing mindful eating, incorporating sustainable protein sources, and prioritizing whole, unprocessed foods, we can support our own health while minimizing the environmental impact of our dietary choices. Embracing sustainable nutrition is not only beneficial for our own well-being but also contributes to a healthier, more sustainable future for generations to come.

# Chapter8

## Gut-Brain Axis and Mental Health

The gut-brain axis is a bidirectional communication system between the gastrointestinal tract and the brain, playing a crucial role in our overall well-being, including mental health. This complex network of connections involves various pathways, including neural, hormonal, and immune mechanisms. In recent years, researchers have uncovered compelling evidence of the significant influence of the gut microbiota on mental health and the development of psychiatric disorders.

The gut microbiota refers to the trillions of microorganisms residing in our digestive system. These microorganisms, primarily bacteria, play a pivotal role in maintaining a healthy gut-brain axis. They produce neurotransmitters, vitamins, and short-chain fatty acids, which can influence brain function and behavior. Disruptions in the gut microbiota composition, known as dysbiosis, have been linked to various mental health conditions, including anxiety, depression, and even neurodevelopmental disorders like autism spectrum disorder.

Studies have demonstrated a correlation between alterations in gut microbiota diversity and mental health disorders. Imbalances in the gut microbiota can lead to increased inflammation, impaired neurotransmitter production, and altered stress response systems, all of which can contribute to the development and progression of mental health conditions.

Furthermore, the gut microbiota's influence on mental health is closely tied to the immune system. The gut houses a significant portion of our immune cells, and a healthy gut microbiota helps regulate immune responses. Dysbiosis can trigger immune dysregulation and chronic low-grade inflammation, which have been associated with psychiatric disorders. This suggests that maintaining a healthy gut microbiota is essential for both immune and mental health.

Diet plays a crucial role in shaping the gut microbiota and influencing the gut-brain axis. A diet rich in fiber and diverse plant-based foods provides the necessary nutrients for a thriving gut microbiota. Prebiotics, found in foods like onions, garlic, and bananas, serve as fuel for beneficial gut bacteria. Probiotics, live microorganisms found in fermented foods like yogurt and kimchi, can also positively influence the gut microbiota and mental health.

In addition to diet, lifestyle factors such as stress management and sleep have been found to impact the gut-brain axis. Chronic stress can disrupt the gut microbiota composition and compromise gut barrier function, leading to increased permeability (leaky gut) and inflammation. Adequate sleep, on the other hand, supports gut health and enhances the gut-brain axis by promoting healthy immune function and reducing stress.

The emerging field of psychobiotics explores the use of specific bacteria or their metabolites as therapeutic interventions for mental health disorders. Clinical trials have shown promising results in using certain probiotics to alleviate symptoms of depression, anxiety, and stress. While further research is needed, these findings suggest the potential of targeting the gut microbiota to improve mental health outcomes.

Understanding the gut-brain axis has opened up new possibilities for treating mental health conditions through interventions that target the gut microbiota. Lifestyle modifications, including a healthy diet, stress reduction techniques, and prioritizing sleep, can promote a balanced gut microbiota and support mental well-being. Additionally, further research into psychobiotics and microbiota-based therapies may pave the way for innovative treatments for mental health disorders.

In summary, the gut-brain axis plays a crucial role in mental health, and disruptions in the gut microbiota have been linked to various psychiatric conditions. Maintaining a healthy gut microbiota through a balanced diet, stress management, and sufficient sleep is essential for supporting mental well-being. The emerging field of psychobiotics holds promise for future interventions in mental health treatment. By nurturing our gut microbiota, we can enhance the communication between our gut and brain and potentially improve mental health outcomes.

# Chapter 9

## The Impact of Processed Foods and Sugar on Mental Health

The food we consume has a significant impact not only on our physical health but also on our mental well-being. In recent years, there has been growing evidence suggesting that a diet high in processed foods and sugar can negatively affect mental health. In this section, we will explore the relationship between processed foods, sugar, and mental health and highlight the potential consequences of their consumption.

Processed foods are typically high in added sugars, unhealthy fats, and artificial additives, while lacking essential nutrients. These foods include fast food, packaged snacks, sugary drinks, and pre-packaged meals. Research has indicated a strong association between a diet high in processed foods and an increased risk of mental health disorders, including depression and anxiety.

One of the reasons for this connection is the impact of processed foods on inflammation in the body. Processed foods, particularly those high in unhealthy fats and added sugars, can trigger a state of chronic low-grade inflammation. Inflammation is known to contribute to the development and progression of mental health conditions. It can affect neurotransmitter production, disrupt the balance of hormones and impact the functioning of the brain.

Moreover, consuming excessive amounts of sugar, commonly found in processed foods, can have detrimental effects on mental health. Sugar consumption leads to rapid spikes in blood sugar levels, followed by crashes, which can cause mood swings, irritability, and fatigue. Over time, a diet high in sugar may contribute to chronic inflammation and impair the brain's ability to regulate emotions and manage stress.

Another important factor to consider is the impact of processed foods on the gut microbiota. The gut microbiota plays a crucial role in regulating brain function and mental health. Research has shown that a diet high in processed foods can negatively affect the diversity and balance of gut bacteria, leading to dysbiosis. Dysbiosis has been associated with mental health disorders, as imbalances in gut bacteria can influence neurotransmitter production and inflammation.

Furthermore, the addictive nature of processed foods and sugar can contribute to poor mental health outcomes. Studies have suggested that the consumption of highly processed foods and sugar can activate reward pathways in the brain, similar to addictive substances. This can lead to cravings, binge-eating, and a cycle of poor dietary choices, which can negatively impact mental well-being and contribute to the development of disordered eating patterns.

Fortunately, making dietary changes can have a positive impact on mental health. Opting for whole, unprocessed foods instead of processed options can provide essential nutrients and support overall well-being. A diet rich in fruits, vegetables, whole grains, lean proteins, and healthy fats is associated with a lower risk of mental health disorders.

Reducing the intake of added sugars is also crucial. Instead of reaching for sugary snacks and beverages, choosing natural sources of sweetness like fruits can satisfy cravings while providing essential nutrients and fiber. It is important to read food labels carefully, as sugar can be found in surprising amounts in many processed foods, even those that are not perceived as sweet.

In conclusion, the consumption of processed foods and excessive sugar intake can have detrimental effects on mental health. These foods can contribute to inflammation, dysregulation of neurotransmitters, and imbalances in the gut microbiota, all of which can impact mood,

cognition, and overall mental
well-being. By opting for a diet rich in
whole, unprocessed foods and
reducing sugar intake, we can
support our mental health and
promote a more balanced and
positive relationship with food.
Making mindful choices about the
foods we consume can have a
profound impact on our mental
well-being, leading to improved

mood, increased energy levels, and better overall mental health.

# Chapter 10

**Lifestyle Factors and Mental Health**

Our lifestyle choices play a significant role in shaping our mental health and well-being. Certain factors, such as physical activity, sleep, stress management, social connections, and self-care practices, can have a profound impact on our mental well-being. In this section, we will explore the relationship between lifestyle factors and mental health, highlighting their importance in promoting overall psychological well-being.

Regular physical activity has been consistently associated with better mental health outcomes. Engaging in exercise releases endorphins, which are natural mood boosters. Physical activity can reduce symptoms of depression and anxiety, improve self-esteem, and enhance cognitive function. Whether it's going for a walk, practicing yoga, or participating in team sports, finding enjoyable ways to incorporate movement into our daily lives can significantly benefit our mental well-being.

Sleep is another vital lifestyle factor that influences mental health. Sufficient, high-quality sleep is essential for proper brain function and emotional regulation. Chronic sleep deprivation has been linked to increased risks of developing mental health disorders, including depression and anxiety. Establishing a regular sleep schedule, creating a relaxing bedtime routine, and ensuring a comfortable sleep environment are essential practices for promoting optimal mental well-being.

Stress management is crucial for maintaining good mental health. Chronic stress can contribute to the development and exacerbation of various mental health conditions. Engaging in stress-reducing activities, such as mindfulness meditation,

deep breathing exercises, or
engaging in hobbies and activities
that bring joy and relaxation, can help
mitigate the negative impact of
stress on mental well-being. Building
resilience and developing healthy
coping mechanisms are also
important aspects of stress
management.

Social connections and a supportive
social network are vital for our

mental health. Building and maintaining meaningful relationships can provide emotional support, reduce feelings of loneliness and isolation, and improve overall mental well-being. Engaging in social activities, joining clubs or groups that share similar interests, and fostering positive relationships with friends, family, and community members can significantly contribute to our mental health and happiness.

Self-care practices are essential for nurturing our mental well-being. Taking time for ourselves, engaging in activities we enjoy, and prioritizing self-care can help reduce stress and improve overall mental health. This can include activities such as practicing mindfulness, engaging in creative pursuits, setting boundaries, and engaging in activities that promote relaxation and self-reflection. Self-care is a personal journey, and finding practices that resonate with us individually is key.

Additionally, nutrition and a healthy diet play a crucial role in supporting mental health. Consuming a balanced diet that includes whole, nutrient-dense foods can provide the necessary nutrients for optimal brain function. Certain nutrients, such as omega-3 fatty acids, B vitamins, and antioxidants, have been linked to improved mental well-being. Prioritizing a varied diet that includes fruits, vegetables, whole grains, lean proteins, and healthy fats can support both our physical and mental health.

In conclusion, lifestyle factors have a significant impact on our mental health and well-being. Engaging in regular physical activity, prioritizing quality sleep, managing stress effectively, nurturing social connections, practicing self-care, and maintaining a balanced diet can all contribute to better mental health outcomes. These lifestyle choices support our overall psychological well-being, promote resilience, and enhance our ability to cope with life's challenges. By adopting positive lifestyle practices, we can take proactive steps towards cultivating good mental health and enjoying a more fulfilling and satisfying life.

# NOTE

It's important to note that the information provided in this eBook is intended for general informational purposes only and should not be considered a substitute for professional medical advice, diagnosis, or treatment.

Before making any significant changes to your diet or starting any new nutritional program, it's always advisable to consult with a qualified healthcare professional or a registered dietitian who can assess your individual needs and provide personalized guidance.

Every individual is unique, and what works for one person may not work for another. Factors such as underlying medical conditions, medications, allergies, and personal preferences should be taken into consideration when making dietary changes.

Additionally, the information provided in this eBook should not be used to diagnose or treat any specific mental health condition. If you're experiencing mental health concerns, it's crucial to seek professional help from a qualified mental health practitioner.

Remember, achieving optimal mental health involves a multidimensional approach that includes not only nutrition but also other factors such as exercise, sleep, stress management, and social support. It's important to address these aspects holistically for comprehensive mental well-being.